RECIPES FOR CANCER PREVENTION 2024

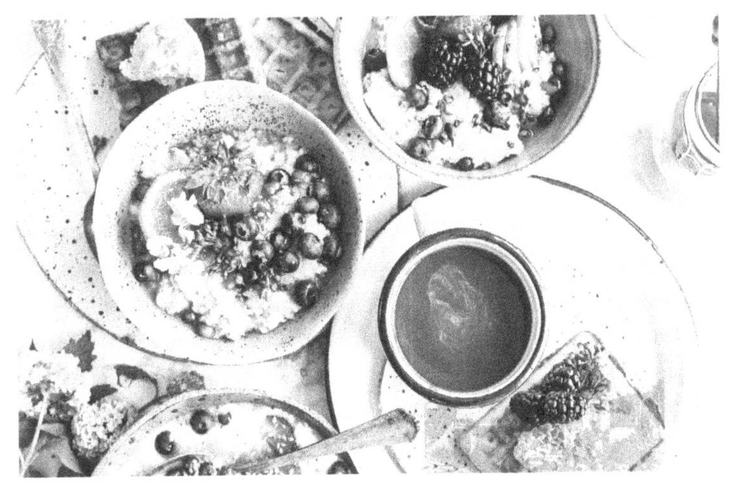

Boost Your Health Naturally with Delicious & Nutritious Meals for Wellness

Misty J. Font

1

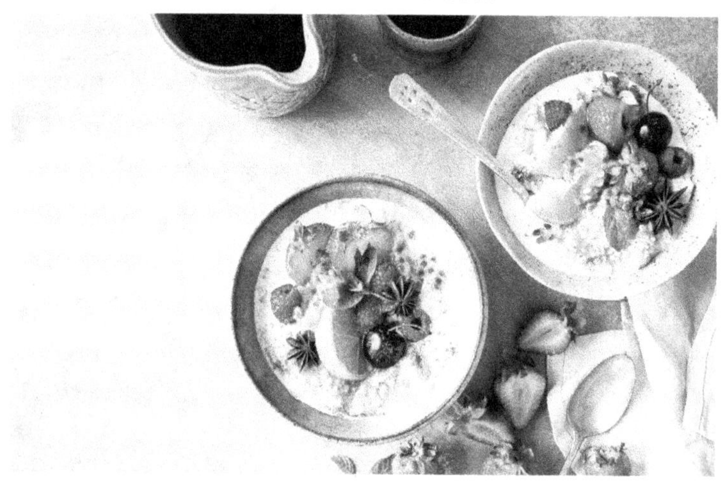

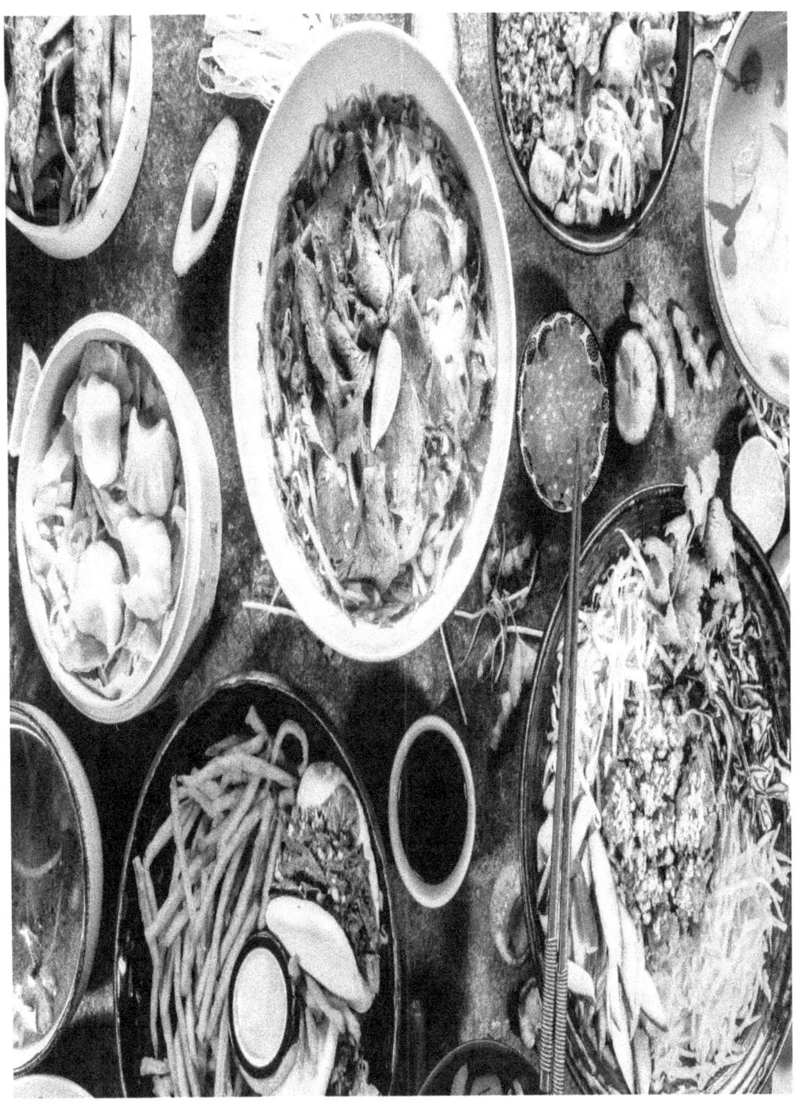

Table of content

CHAPTER 1: INTRODUCTION..................................7

About Cancer Prevention................................ 11

Understanding Cancer and Risk Factors............... 11

Importance of Diet and Nutrition in Cancer Prevention..12

An overview of the role of recipes in cancer prevention... 12

CHAPTER 2: THE SCIENCE BEHIND CANCER-FIGHTING FOODS......................... 14

Phytochemicals and Antioxidants for Cancer Prevention...14

Nutrient-dense Ingredients for a Healthy Diet........15

Including Superfoods in Your Meals..................... 16

CHAPTER 3: BREAKFASTS DELIGHTS....................17

Green Tea Matcha Smoothie Bowl...................... 17

Salmon and Avocado Toast.............................. 18

Turmeric Ginger Smoothie................................19

Broccoli and Feta Omelette.............................. 21

Berry Spinach Salad with Almonds......................22

Cancer-Fighting Smoothie Bowl......................... 23

Quinoa Breakfast Salad....................................25

Ginger-Turmeric Chia Pudding........................... 26

Mushroom Spinach Frittata...............................27

Blueberry Walnut Overnight Oats........................ 29

CHAPTER 4: LUNCH FAVORITE............................31

Grilled Chicken and Quinoa Salad.......................31

Salmon and Asparagus Stir-Fry...........................32

Mediterranean Chickpea Salad........................... 34

Vegetarian Lentil Soup.................................35

Tuna Avocado Wrap.................................. 37

Quinoa Stuffed Bell Peppers................................. 38

Broccoli Walnut Pasta...39

Curried Chickpea Salad Wraps............................ 41

Grilled Vegetable Quinoa Bowl............................. 45

CHAPTER 5: NOURISHING DINNER......................... 47

Grilled salmon with roasted vegetables................. 47

This flavorful dish combines grilled salmon with a medley of roasted vegetables to create a delicious and cancer-preventive dinner option..................... 47

Quinoa Stuffed Bell Peppers.............................. 48

Mushroom Lentil Bolognese Pasta....................... 50

Grilled Chicken and Veggie Skewers.....................51

Roasted Butternut Squash Soup........................... 53

Turmeric Spiced Chickpea Curry.......................... 54

Baked Stuffed Sweet Potatoes............................. 56

Veggie Stir-Fry with Tofu....................................58

Lemon Herb Grilled Chicken................................60

Vegetarian Lentil Shepherd's Pie.........................61

CHAPTER 6: SNACKS AND SIDES......................... 64

Avocado and Chickpea Salad................................64

Roasted Beet Hummus.......................................65

Quinoa and Black Bean Stuffed Bell Peppers........ 67

Greek Yogurt Veggie Dip................................... 68

Crispy Baked Kale Chips.................................... 70

Coconut Mango Chia Pudding.............................71

Turmeric Roasted Cauliflower..............................73

Spinach and Feta Stuffed Mushrooms.................. 74

Baked Sweet Potato Fries................................... 76

Mediterranean Chickpea Salad............................ 77

CHAPTER 7: DESSERTS AND TREATS.....................80

Berry Chia Seed Pudding.................................... 80

Dark Chocolate Avocado Mousse......................... 81

Turmeric Golden Milk Popsicles........................... 82

Matcha Green Tea Nice Cream............................ 84

Oatmeal Raisin Energy Bites...............................85

Coconut Almond Bliss Balls................................ 86

Pumpkin Spice Chia Pudding............................... 87

Blueberry Yogurt Parfait.................................... 89

Cinnamon Apple Crisp....................................... 90

Coconut Mango Sorbet...................................... 91

CHAPTER8 : BONUS 7-DAY MEAL PLANNING........94

CONCLUSION...97

Additional Resources..97

CHAPTER 1:
INTRODUCTION

Merry had always had a passion for cooking and trying new recipes. Her passion for creating delectable dishes served as both an outlet for her creativity and a source of nourishment for herself and her loved ones. Merry's interest in the relationship between food and health grew as she learned more about the culinary arts.

Merry came across a cookbook, "Cancer Prevention Recipes: Nourishing Dishes for a Healthy Lifestyle," while browsing through a bookstore. Merry was intrigued by the title and the promise of recipes that could potentially help with cancer prevention, so she decided to buy the book and read its contents.

Merry was captivated by the cookbook's vibrant photographs of colorful dishes, as well as the detailed descriptions of ingredients and cooking methods. The recipes in the book were not only delicious, but also included cancer-fighting ingredients like antioxidant-rich berries, turmeric, green tea, and nuts.

Merry decided to embark on a culinary journey guided by the Cancer Prevention Cookbook after being inspired by the recipes' potential to not only satisfy her taste buds but also contribute to her overall well-being. She resolved to prioritize her health and investigate the potential of food as a preventive measure against diseases such as cancer.

Merry began experimenting with the cookbook's recipes, starting with simple but flavorful dishes such as Berry Chia Seed Pudding and Dark Chocolate Avocado Mousse. She enjoyed the process of preparing these dishes, savoring each bite with a renewed appreciation for the nourishment they provided to her body.

Merry noticed that as she continued to experiment with the cookbook's recipes, her energy levels and overall health improved. She felt more energized and rejuvenated after incorporating nutrient-dense ingredients into her meals.

Merry's favorite recipe in the cookbook was the Turmeric Golden Milk Popsicles. The refreshing popsicles infused with turmeric, ginger, and coconut milk became a freezer staple, providing a delicious and guilt-free summer treat.

Merry also enjoyed making batches of Matcha Green Tea Nice Cream and Oatmeal Raisin Energy Bites for quick and filling snacks throughout the day. These nutritious treats not only satisfied her cravings but also gave her a boost of energy and vitality.

Merry's journey with the Cancer Prevention Cookbook gave her a new sense of empowerment in the kitchen. She realized she had the ability to nourish her body and protect her health by choosing the foods she ate.

Merry felt a deep sense of gratitude for the role that food played in supporting her health as she continued to explore the recipes in the cookbook and adopt a holistic well-being lifestyle. Merry took pleasure in knowing that with each meal she prepared, she was taking proactive steps toward cancer prevention and overall wellness.

When Merry incorporated the Cancer Prevention Cookbook principles into her daily routine, she discovered not only a newfound passion for cooking, but also a profound appreciation for food's transformative power. Merry embarked on a journey towards vibrant health and well-being, one delicious dish at a time, thanks to the cookbook's guidance.

About Cancer Prevention

Cancer. The mere mention of this word can instill fear, uncertainty, and a feeling of vulnerability. It is a disease that has touched the lives of millions, causing pain and suffering for individuals and families all over the world. But, despite the darkness of cancer, there is hope: hope in the power of prevention.

Understanding Cancer and Risk Factors

To effectively combat cancer, we must first comprehend it. Cancer is a complex disease characterized by the uncontrolled proliferation and spread of abnormal cells throughout the body. It can take many forms, affecting various organs and systems. While genetics play a role in cancer development, environmental and lifestyle factors also have a significant impact.

Importance of Diet and Nutrition in Cancer Prevention

Diet is one of the most powerful tools we have in the fight against cancer. According to research, certain foods and nutrients can help lower the risk of developing cancer and even inhibit the growth of existing cancer cells. A diet high in fruits, vegetables, whole grains, lean proteins, and healthy fats can provide the body with the nutrients it needs to build a strong immune system and maintain cellular health.

An overview of the role of recipes in cancer prevention

Recipes are more than just meal preparation instructions; they also serve as a gateway to health and wellness. By carefully selecting ingredients and preparing balanced meals, we can harness the power of food to prevent cancer and promote overall health. This chapter will look at how recipes can be a useful and delicious tool in the fight against cancer.

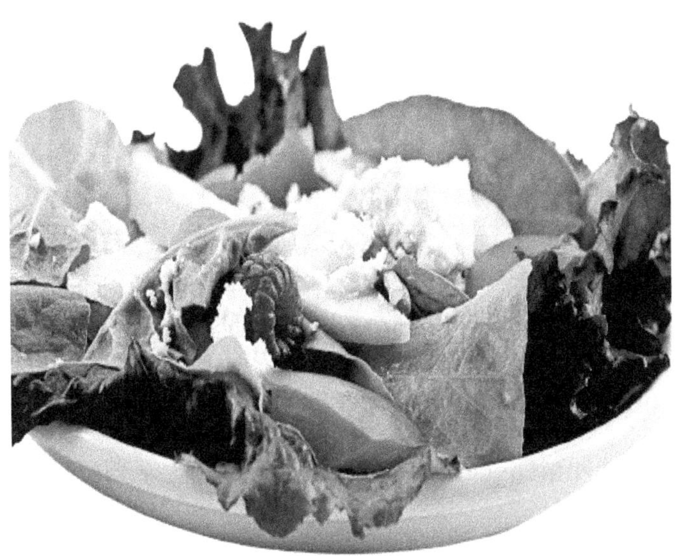

CHAPTER 2: THE SCIENCE BEHIND CANCER-FIGHTING FOODS

In the fight against cancer, knowledge is power. Understanding the science behind cancer-fighting foods allows us to make more informed decisions that benefit our health and well-being. This chapter will delve into the fascinating world of phytochemicals, antioxidants, nutrient-dense foods, and superfoods, looking at how these elements play an important role in cancer prevention.

Phytochemicals and Antioxidants for Cancer Prevention

Phytochemicals are natural compounds found in plant-based foods that have been shown to have potent anticancer properties. These bioactive substances work in tandem with antioxidants to neutralize harmful free radicals in the body, which can damage cells and contribute to cancer growth. We can harness the protective effects of phytochemical-rich foods like berries, cruciferous vegetables, and herbs in our diet to lower our risk of cancer.

Antioxidants, on the other hand, are molecules that fight oxidative stress and inflammation in the body. They play an important role in cell protection and immune system function. Antioxidant-rich foods, such as colorful fruits, leafy greens, nuts, and seeds, can help our bodies defend against cancer-causing agents while also promoting overall health.

Nutrient-dense Ingredients for a Healthy Diet

Maintaining a nutrient-dense diet rich in vitamins, minerals, and other bioactive compounds is an important part of cancer prevention. By eating whole, minimally processed foods, we can ensure that our bodies receive the nutrients they require to function properly and avoid disease. Including a variety of nutrient-dense ingredients, such as whole grains, lean proteins, healthy fats, and dairy alternatives, can help us lay a solid foundation for good health and lower our risk of cancer.

Including Superfoods in Your Meals

Superfoods are nutritional powerhouses that provide a variety of health benefits, including cancer prevention. Superfoods, which range from vibrant berries bursting with antioxidants to leafy greens brimming with phytochemicals, can be a delicious and powerful addition to our diets. By incorporating these nutrient-dense ingredients into our recipes, we can boost our diet's nutritional value while also supporting our bodies' natural cancer defenses.

CHAPTER 3: BREAKFASTS DELIGHTS

Green Tea Matcha Smoothie Bowl

This antioxidant-rich smoothie bowl combines green tea matcha, creamy coconut milk, and fresh fruits for a refreshing and cancer-preventive breakfast.

Serving Size: One.

Prep time: 5 minutes.

Cooking time: 0 minutes.

The ingredients are:

- One teaspoon of green tea matcha powder.
- 1/2 cup coconut milk
- One banana.
- A handful of spinach leaves.
- Toppings include sliced kiwi, shredded coconut, and chia seeds.

Instructions:

1. Blend together the green tea matcha powder, coconut milk, banana, and spinach leaves.
2. Blend until smooth and creamy.
3. Transfer the smoothie to a bowl and top with sliced kiwi, shredded coconut, and chia seeds.
4. Savor this energizing and immune-boosting green tea matcha smoothie bowl.

Salmon and Avocado Toast

This savory breakfast toast contains omega-3 rich salmon and creamy avocado, which are essential nutrients for cancer prevention and overall health.

Serving Size: 1–2 slices

Prep time: 10 minutes.

Cook time: 5 minutes

The ingredients are:

2 slices of whole grain bread - Smoked salmon slices.

one ripe avocado, mashed

Lemon Juice

Fresh dill or chives as garnish

Instructions:

1. Toast the whole-grain bread until golden brown.
2. Spread the mashed avocado on the toast, then drizzle with lemon juice.
3. Garnish with smoked salmon slices.
4. Sprinkle with fresh dill or chives.
5. Make this delicious and nutrient-dense salmon and avocado toast for a filling breakfast.

Turmeric Ginger Smoothie

This anti-inflammatory smoothie combines turmeric, ginger, and citrus fruits for a zesty and immune-boosting start to the day.

Serving Size: One.

__Prep time:__ 5 minutes.

__Cooking time:__ 0 minutes.

__The ingredients are:__

- One teaspoon of turmeric powder.
- 1 inch of fresh ginger, peeled
- Juice from 1 orange
- A handful of pineapple chunks.
- Water or coconut water.

__Instructions:__

1. Blend together the turmeric powder, fresh ginger, orange juice, pineapple chunks, and coconut water.
2. Blend until smooth and thoroughly combined.
3. Pour the turmeric ginger smoothie into a glass and enjoy this colorful, immune-boosting breakfast option.

Broccoli and Feta Omelette

This protein-packed omelette is filled with nutrient-dense broccoli and tangy feta cheese, making it a delicious and cancer-preventive breakfast option.

Serving Size: One.

Prep time: 10 minutes.

Cook time: 10 minutes

Ingredients:

- Two eggs.
- Steamed broccoli florets with feta cheese crumbles.
- Add salt and pepper to taste. - Cook with olive oil.

Instructions:

1. In a bowl, whisk together the eggs, salt, and pepper until well combined.

2. Heat the olive oil in a skillet over medium heat.

3. Place the steamed broccoli florets in the skillet.

4. Pour the whisked eggs over the broccoli.

5. Sprinkle the feta cheese crumbles on top.

6. Cook the omelette until set and golden brown on both sides.

7. Serve this flavorful broccoli and feta omelette hot for a healthy breakfast.

Berry Spinach Salad with Almonds

Combine antioxidant-rich berries, nutrient-dense spinach, and crunchy almonds for a refreshing and cancer-preventing breakfast.

Serving Size: One.

Prep time: 10 minutes, cooking time: 0 minutes.

Ingredients:

- Baby spinach leaves

- Mixed berries (e.g., strawberries, blueberries, raspberries)
- Sliced almonds.
- Balsamic vinaigrette dressing.

Instructions:

1. In a bowl, combine the baby spinach leaves, mixed berries, and sliced almonds.
2. Toss the salad with the balsamic vinaigrette dressing.
3. Serve this colorful and nutrient-dense berry spinach salad as a light and refreshing breakfast.

Cancer-Fighting Smoothie Bowl

This superfood smoothie bowl contains cancer-fighting ingredients such as berries, kale, and nuts to promote overall health and well-being.

Serving size: one - Preparation time: five minutes

Cooking time: 0 minutes.

Ingredients:

- Kale leave Mixed
- berries (e.g. blueberries, raspberries)
- Walnuts.
- Coconut water or almond milk.

Toppings:

- sliced banana,
- chia seeds,
- and granola.

Instructions:

1. In a blender, combine kale, mixed berries, walnuts, and coconut water or almond milk.
2. Blend until smooth and creamy.
3. Pour the smoothie into a bowl, then top with sliced banana, chia seeds, and granola.
4. For a nutritious breakfast, try this cancer-fighting smoothie bowl.

Quinoa Breakfast Salad

Protein-rich quinoa, avocado, tomatoes, and leafy greens make for a satisfying and cancer-preventive morning meal.

Serving Size: One.

Prep time: 15 minutes.

Cook time: 15 minutes

Ingredients:

- 1/2 cup cooked quinoa,
- 1/2 diced avocado,
- halved cherry tomatoes,
- mixed greens (arugula or spinach),
- and lemon vinaigrette dressing.

Instructions:

1. In a bowl, combine the cooked quinoa, diced avocado, cherry tomatoes, and mixed greens.

2. Drizzle with lemon vinaigrette and toss to combine.

3. Serve this protein-rich quinoa breakfast salad for a nutritious and filling start to the day.

Ginger-Turmeric Chia Pudding

This anti-inflammatory chia pudding with ginger and turmeric boosts immunity and can prevent cancer.

Serving Size: One.

Prep time is 5 minutes (plus chilling time).

Cooking time: 0 minutes.

Ingredients:

- 2 tablespoons chia seeds,
- 1/2 teaspoon ground ginger,
- and 1/2 teaspoon ground turmeric.
- Coconut or almond milk.
- Sliced mango or berries as a topping

Instructions:

1. In a jar or container, mix together the chia seeds, ground ginger, ground turmeric, and coconut or almond milk.
2. Stir thoroughly to combine all ingredients.
3. Cover the jar or container and chill for at least two hours, preferably overnight, to allow the chia seeds to thicken.
4. Serve this ginger-turmeric chia pudding with sliced mango or berries for a delicious and nutritious breakfast.

Mushroom Spinach Frittata

This protein-rich breakfast with mushrooms, spinach, and eggs promotes cancer prevention and overall health.

Servings: 1-2.

Prep time: 10 minutes.

Cook time: 20 minutes

Ingredients:

- sliced mushrooms,
- baby spinach leaves,
- and four eggs.
- Grated Parmesan cheese is optional.
- Season with salt and pepper to taste.

Instructions:

1. Heat the oven to 350°F (180°C).
2. In an oven-safe skillet, cook the mushrooms until golden brown.
3. Cook the baby spinach leaves until wilted.
4. In a bowl, whisk together the eggs, salt, and pepper.
5. Pour the egg mixture onto the mushrooms and spinach in the skillet.
6. Cook on the stovetop for a few minutes, until the edges begin to set.
7. If using, sprinkle grated Parmesan cheese on top and place the skillet in the oven.

8. Bake for 10-15 minutes, or until the frittata is firm and cooked through.

9. Serve this mushroom spinach frittata warm for a hearty breakfast.

Blueberry Walnut Overnight Oats

Infused with antioxidant-rich blueberries, omega-3-rich walnuts, and fiber-packed oats, this breakfast option is both convenient and cancer-preventive.

Servings: 1-2.

Prep time is 5 minutes (plus chilling time).

Cooking time: 0 minutes.

Ingredients:

- 1/2 cup rolled oats
- Fresh or frozen blueberries
- Chopped walnuts
- Almond milk or Greek yogurt.
- Add maple syrup or honey for sweetness.

Instructions:

1. In a jar or container, combine rolled oats, blueberries, chopped walnuts, almond milk or Greek yogurt, and desired sweetener.

2. Stir thoroughly to combine all ingredients.

3. Cover the jar or container and refrigerate overnight, or at least four hours.

4. In the morning, stir the blueberry walnut overnight oats thoroughly before serving this deliciously nutritious breakfast.

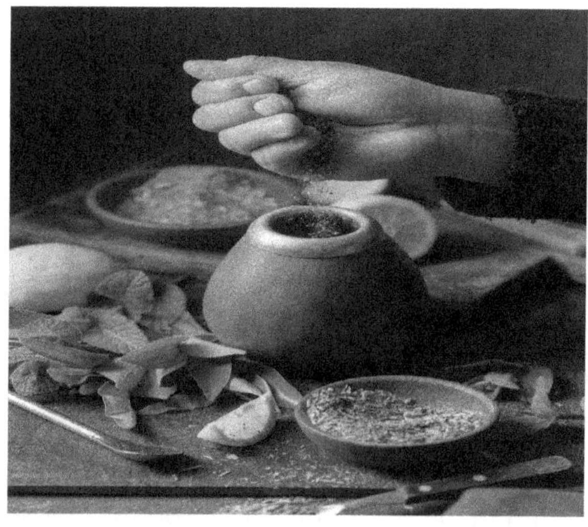

CHAPTER 4: LUNCH FAVORITE

Grilled Chicken and Quinoa Salad

This protein-rich salad with colorful vegetables is a satisfying and cancer-preventive lunch option.

Serving Size: One.

Preparation time is 15 minutes, followed by cooking time of 15 minutes.

The ingredients are:

- 4 oz grilled chicken breast (sliced)
- 1/2 cup cooked quinoa.
- Mixed greens (spinach or arugula)
- Halved cherry tomatoes - Sliced cucumber
- Red bell pepper, diced
- Balsamic vinaigrette dressing.

Instructions:

1. In a bowl, combine the grilled chicken, cooked quinoa, mixed greens, cherry tomatoes, cucumber, and red bell pepper.
2. Toss the salad with the balsamic vinaigrette dressing.
3. Make this flavorful and nutrient-dense grilled chicken and quinoa salad for a balanced lunch.

Salmon and Asparagus Stir-Fry

A healthy and cancer-preventive lunch option with omega-3-rich salmon, fiber-packed asparagus, and a flavorful sauce.

Serving size: two.

Prep time: 10 minutes.

Cook time: 15 minutes

The ingredients are:

- 8-ounce salmon fillet cut into cubes.

- Trim and cut 1 bunch of asparagus into pieces.
- Mince garlic.
- Soy Sauce
- Ingredients include grated ginger and sesame oil.

Instructions:

1. In a skillet, heat the sesame oil over medium heat.
2. Sauté the minced garlic and grated ginger until fragrant.
3. Cook the salmon cubes until browned on all sides.
4. Add the asparagus pieces and soy sauce, and stir-fry until tender and crisp.
5. Serve this savory salmon and asparagus stir-fry hot with brown rice for a delicious and cancer-preventing lunch.

Mediterranean Chickpea Salad

This salad contains protein-rich chickpeas, colorful vegetables, and tangy feta cheese, making it a refreshing and cancer-preventive lunch option.

Serves 2 people - Takes 15 minutes to prepare.

Cooking time: 0 minutes.

Ingredients:

- 1 can rinsed and drained chickpeas - Halved cherry tomatoes
- Diced cucumber
- Thinly sliced red onion
- Kalamata olives
- Feta cheese crumbles
- Lemon vinaigrette dressing.

Instructions:

1. In a bowl, combine the chickpeas, cherry tomatoes, cucumber, red onion, Kalamata olives, and feta cheese crumbles.

2. Drizzle with lemon vinaigrette and toss to combine.

3. Chill this Mediterranean chickpea salad for a flavorful and nutritious lunch.

Vegetarian Lentil Soup

This hearty soup with protein-rich lentils, colorful vegetables, and aromatic spices is a comforting and cancer-preventive meal option.

Serving size: four.

Prep time: 10 minutes, cooking time: 30 minutes.

Ingredients:

- 1 cup dried lentils,
- rinsed.
- diced carrots,
- chopped celery,

- diced onion,

- and minced garlic.

- Vegetable broth with cumin, turmeric, and paprika.

Instructions:

1. In a pot, cook the diced onion and garlic until fragrant.

2. Cook the diced carrots and celery until slightly softened.

3. Mix in the rinsed lentils, vegetable broth, cumin, turmeric, and paprika.

4. Simmer for 20-25 minutes, until the lentils are tender.

5. Serve this vegetarian lentil soup hot with a sprinkle of fresh herbs for a nourishing and cancer-fighting lunch.

Tuna Avocado Wrap

Combine protein-rich tuna, creamy avocado, and crunchy vegetables in a whole grain tortilla for a satisfying and cancer-preventive lunch.

Serving Size: 1–2 wraps

Prep time: 10 minutes.

Cooking time: 0 minutes.

Ingredients:

- Drain canned tuna in water.
- ripe avocado, mashed
- Bell pepper strips (red, yellow, or orange) - Spinach leaves
- Whole grain tortillas

Instructions:

1. Arrange the whole grain tortillas on a flat surface.
2. Spread mashed avocado over each tortilla.

3. Add canned tuna, bell pepper strips, and spinach leaves.

4. Roll the tortillas into wraps and cut in half.

5. Serve these tuna avocado wraps with a side of fresh fruit for a quick and healthy lunch.

Quinoa Stuffed Bell Peppers

A flavorful and nutritious lunch option with protein-rich quinoa, black beans, corn, and spices.

Serving Size: 2 to 4 peppers

Prep time: 20 minutes, cooking time: 30 minutes.

Ingredients:

- halved and seeded bell peppers of any color, as well as cooked quinoa.

- Black beans (drained and rinsed)

- Corn kernels, fresh or frozen.

- salsa or diced tomatoes

- Mexican spices (cumin and chili powder)

Instructions:

1. Preheat your oven to 375°F (190°C).

2. In a bowl, combine the cooked quinoa, black beans, corn kernels, salsa or diced tomatoes, and Mexican spices.

3. Stuff the quinoa mixture into the halved bell peppers.

4. Transfer the stuffed bell peppers to a baking dish and cover with foil.

5. Bake for 25-30 minutes, until the peppers are tender.

6. Serve these quinoa-stuffed bell peppers hot with a dollop of Greek yogurt or avocado for a nutritious and delicious lunch.

Broccoli Walnut Pasta

This nutrient-dense pasta dish combines whole grain noodles, roasted broccoli, omega-3-rich walnuts, and a light lemon garlic sauce for a flavorful and cancer-preventive lunch.

Serving size: two.

Prep time: 15 minutes, cooking time: 20 minutes.

Ingredients:

- whole grain pasta,
- broccoli florets,
- chopped walnuts,
- and minced garlic cloves.
- Combine lemon juice and zest with olive oil.

Instructions:

1. Cook whole grain pasta according to the package directions.
2. Toss the broccoli florets in olive oil and roast in the oven until tender.
3. In a skillet, cook the minced garlic in olive oil until fragrant.
4. Stir in the cooked pasta, roasted broccoli, chopped walnuts, lemon juice, and zest to the skillet.

5. Toss everything until thoroughly combined.

6. For a satisfying lunch, serve this broccoli walnut pasta hot with a sprinkle of Parmesan or nutritional yeast.

Curried Chickpea Salad Wraps

These flavorful wraps feature spiced chickpea salad with crunchy vegetables wrapped in whole grain tortillas for a satisfying and cancer-preventive lunch option, perfect for on-the-go meals.

Serving Size: 2–4 wraps

Prep time: 15 minutes.

Cooking time: 0 minutes.

Ingredients:

- Canned chickpeas (drained and rinsed)
- finely chopped red onion and diced bell pepper (any color).
- Cucumber diced

For Dressing:

- Greek yogurt.

- Curry Powder

- Lemon Juice

Additional ingredients

- Whole grain tortillas.

- Spinach leaves

- Sliced tomatoes

- Sliced avocado

Instructions:

1. In a large mixing bowl, combine drained chickpeas, red onion, bell pepper, and cucumber.

2. To prepare the dressing, combine Greek yogurt, curry powder, and lemon juice in a separate small bowl.

3. Pour the dressing over the chickpea mixture and toss to coat evenly.

4. Lay out whole grain tortillas and place spinach leaves on each one.

5. Divide the chickpea salad among the tortillas, then top with sliced tomatoes and avocado.

6. Roll each tortilla tightly into wraps and cut in half if desired.

7. Enjoy these curried chickpea salad wraps for a flavorful and nutritious lunch!

Vegan Lentil Tacos

These plant-based tacos contain protein-rich lentils, avocado, and fresh vegetables, making them both delicious and cancer-preventive.

Service Size: Makes approximately 8 tacos.

*Prep Time:*15 minutes.

*Cook Time:*20 minutes

Ingredients:

- 1 cup dried green or brown lentils.
- Taco Seasoning
- Corn tortillas
- Avocado slices
- Shredded lettuce

- Diced tomatoes.

- Diced red onions

- Cilantro leaves.

- Lime wedges.

Instructions:

1. Cook the lentils according to package directions, then season with taco seasoning to taste.

2. Heat the corn tortillas in a skillet or microwave.

3. Fill each tortilla with lentils, then top with avocado, lettuce, tomatoes, onion, cilantro, and lime juice.

4. Top these vegan lentil tacos with your favorite salsa or hot sauce for a tasty and nutritious meal!

Grilled Vegetable Quinoa Bowl

This colorful bowl with grilled vegetables, protein-packed quinoa, and creamy avocado is a nutritious and cancer-preventive lunch option.

Service Size: Makes about servings.

*Preparation Time:*minutes.

*Cook Time:*minutes

Ingredients:

- Cooked Quinoa
- Grilled vegetables (bell peppers, zucchini, and mushrooms).
- One-half cherry tomatoes
- Sliced avocado
- Balsamic vinaigrette dressing.

Instructions:

1. In a bowl, combine cooked quinoa, grilled vegetables, cherry tomatoes, and sliced avocado.

2. Drizzle with balsamic vinaigrette dressing and gently toss.

3. Serve this grilled vegetable quinoa bowl warm or at room temperature for a filling and nutritious lunch.

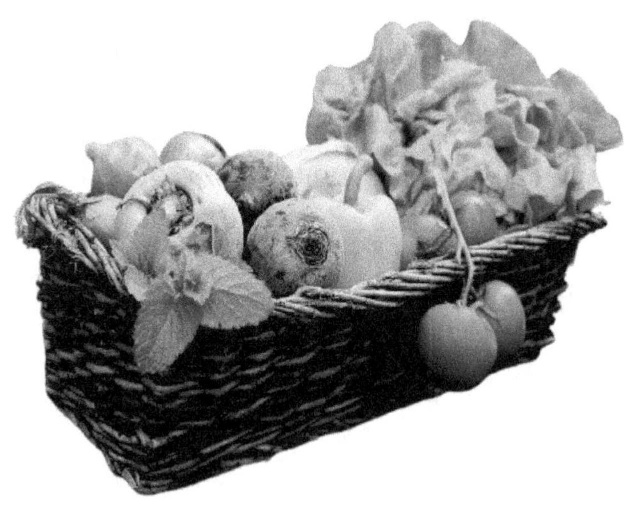

CHAPTER 5: NOURISHING DINNER

Grilled salmon with roasted vegetables

This flavorful dish combines grilled salmon with a medley of roasted vegetables to create a delicious and cancer-preventive dinner option.

Serves 2 people - Takes 15 minutes to prepare - Cooks for 20 minutes

Ingredients:

- Two salmon fillets - Bell peppers, zucchini, and cherry tomatoes
- Olive Oil
- Garlic powder,
- paprika,
- salt, and pepper.

Instructions:

1. Preheat the grill, then season the salmon fillets with garlic powder, paprika, salt, and pepper.
2. Grill the salmon until fully cooked.
3. Mix the chopped vegetables with olive oil, salt, and pepper.
4. Roast the vegetables in the oven until they are tender.
5. Pair the grilled salmon with the roasted vegetables for a nutritious and filling dinner.

Quinoa Stuffed Bell Peppers

A flavorful and nutritious dinner option with protein-rich quinoa, black beans, corn, and spices.

Serving size: four.

Prep time: 20 minutes, cooking time: 30 minutes.

Ingredients:

- Halved and seeded bell peppers of any color

- Cooked quinoa

- Drained and rinsed black beans.

- Corn kernels, fresh or frozen.

- salsa or diced tomatoes

- Mexican spices (cumin and chili powder)

Instructions:

1. Preheat your oven to 375°F (190°C).

2. In a bowl, combine the cooked quinoa, black beans, corn kernels, salsa or diced tomatoes, and Mexican spices.

3. Stuff the quinoa mixture into the halved bell peppers.

4. Transfer the stuffed bell peppers to a baking dish and cover with foil.

5. Bake for 25-30 minutes, until the peppers are tender.

6. Serve these quinoa-stuffed bell peppers hot with a dollop of Greek yogurt or avocado for a nutritious and delicious dinner.

Mushroom Lentil Bolognese Pasta

A hearty vegetarian pasta dish with a rich mushroom and lentil bolognese sauce served over whole grain noodles is a comforting and cancer-preventive dinner option.

Serving size: four.

Prep time: 15 minutes.

Cook time: 30 minutes

Ingredients:

- include whole grain pasta, diced mushrooms, and cooked lentils.
- diced onion and minced garlic.
- Tomato Sauce
- Italian herbs (basil and oregano) -

Instructions:

1. Cook whole grain pasta according to the package directions.

2. In a skillet, cook the diced onion and minced garlic until soft.

3. Cook the diced mushrooms until browned.

4. Add the cooked lentils, tomato sauce, and Italian herbs.

5. Simmer the bolognese sauce for approximately 20-25 minutes.

6. Pour the mushroom lentil bolognese over the cooked pasta for a flavorful and nutritious dinner.

Grilled Chicken and Veggie Skewers

These colorful skewers feature marinated grilled chicken and a variety of fresh vegetables, making them a delicious and cancer-preventive dinner option.

Serving size: four.

Prep time: 20 minutes.

Cook time: 15 minutes

Ingredients:

- Cut chicken breast into cubes
- Bell peppers,
- cherry tomatoes,
- zucchini,
- and red onions
- Olive Oil
- Lemon juice, garlic, dried herbs (rosemary and thyme)

Instructions:

1. In a bowl, combine olive oil, lemon juice, minced garlic, and dried herbs.
2. Let the chicken cubes marinate in the mixture for at least 15 minutes.
3. Thread marinated chicken and vegetables onto skewers.
4. Grill the skewers until the chicken is fully cooked and the vegetables are tender.

5. For a complete dinner, serve these grilled chicken and vegetable skewers hot with quinoa or brown rice.

Roasted Butternut Squash Soup

This creamy My soup combines roasted butternut squash with warming spices for a comforting and cancer-preventing dinner option ideal for cooler evenings.

Serving size: four.

Prep time: 15 minutes, cooking time: 45 minutes.

Ingredients:

- Peeled and cubed butternut squash Chopped onion
- Minced garlic cloves.
- Vegetable broth - Coconut milk.
- Cinnamon, nutmeg, and cayenne pepper

Instructions:

1. Preheat your oven to 400°F (200°C).

2. Toss the cubed butternut squash with olive oil and place it on a baking sheet.

3. Roast the squash in the oven until soft and caramelized.

4. In a pot, cook the chopped onion and garlic until translucent.

5. Combine the roasted butternut squash, vegetable broth, coconut milk, and spices in the pot.

6. Simmer the soup for approximately 20-25 minutes.

7. Blend the soup until it's smooth and creamy.

8. For a cozy dinner, serve this roasted butternut squash soup hot, garnished with fresh herbs.

Turmeric Spiced Chickpea Curry

Simmer protein-packed chickpeas in a turmeric-spiced coconut milk sauce with colorful vegetables for a flavorful and cancer-preventive dinner.

Serving size: four.

Prep time: 15 minutes, cooking time: 30 minutes.

Ingredients:

- Drained and rinsed canned chickpeas Diced onion
- Diced bell peppers
- Cauliflower florets
- Coconut milk.
- Turmeric,
- cumin,
- and coriander

Instructions:

1. In a pot, cook the diced onion until softened.
2. Cook the diced bell peppers and cauliflower florets until slightly tender.

3. Mix in the drained chickpeas, coconut milk, turmeric, cumin, and coriander.

4. Allow the curry to simmer for 20-25 minutes, or until the vegetables are tender.

5. For a satisfying and nutritious dinner, serve this turmeric-spiced chickpea curry hot over cooked brown rice or quinoa.

Baked Stuffed Sweet Potatoes

Loaded with black beans, corn, avocado, and spices, these sweet potatoes are a nutrient-dense and satisfying cancer-prevention dinner option.

Serves 4 people - Takes 15 minutes to prepare - Cooks for 45 minutes.

Ingredients:

- for stuffed sweet potatoes include sweet potatoes,
- black beans,
- and corn kernels. Avocado

For seasoning:

- cumin,
- paprika,
- garlic powder
- Season with salt and pepper.

Instructions:

1. Preheat oven to 400°F (200°C).
2. Wash sweet potatoes and pierce them multiple times with a fork.
3. Place sweet potatoes on a baking sheet and bake for a few minutes, or until tender.
4. In a bowl, combine black beans, corn kernels, and avocado.
5. Season the bean mixture with cumin, paprika, garlic powder, salt, and pepper.
6. Split the baked sweet potatoes open and fill with the bean mixture.
7. Serve these baked stuffed sweet potatoes hot for a tasty and nutritious dinner option!

Veggie Stir-Fry with Tofu

This colorful stir-fry with tofu and a variety of fresh vegetables in a savory sauce is a delicious and cancer-preventing dinner option.

Service Size: Makes about servings.

Preparation Time: minutes.

Cook Time: minutes

Ingredients:

- Firm tofu,
- cubed
- Broccoli florets
- Sliced bell peppers
- Sliced carrots
- Soy sauce
- Garlic,minced
- Ginger, freshly grated
- Cornstarch

Instructions:

1. In a wok or large skillet, heat the oil over medium-high heat.

2. Add the tofu cubes and cook until golden brown on all sides.

3. Remove tofu from the wok and set aside.

4. In the same wok, add more oil as needed and stir-fry broccoli, bell peppers, and carrots until tender-crisp.

5. In a small bowl, combine soy sauce, minced garlic, freshly grated ginger, and cornstarch to make the sauce.

6. Pour the sauce over the vegetables in the wok and then add the tofu.

7. Stir-fry all ingredients until

8. Well combined, and the sauce thickens slightly.

9. Serve this veggie stir-fry with tofu hot over cooked brown rice or quinoa for a tasty and nutritious dinner!

Lemon Herb Grilled Chicken

For a delicious and cancer-preventive dinner, marinate this flavorful grilled chicken in lemon juice, fresh herbs, and garlic.

Service Size: Makes about servings.

Preparation Time: minutes.

Cook Time: minutes

Ingredients:

- Chicken Breasts
- Lemon Juice
- Olive oil.
- Garlic,minced
- Fresh herbs (rosemary and parsley)
- Salt and pepper.

Instructions:

1. In a mixing bowl, combine lemon juice, olive oil, minced garlic, fresh herbs, salt, and pepper to make the marinade.

2. Place chicken breasts in a shallow dish or resealable plastic bag and pour marinade over them.

3. Marinate the chicken in the refrigerator for an hour or overnight.

4. Preheat the grill to medium-high heat and grill the chicken breasts until cooked through.

5. Serve this lemon herb grilled chicken hot with roasted vegetables or salad for a delicious and cancer-preventive dinner!

Vegetarian Lentil Shepherd's Pie

This comforting shepherd's pie contains protein-rich lentils, tender vegetables, and creamy mashed potatoes, making it a delicious and cancer-preventive dinner option.

Service Size: Makes about servings.

Preparation Time: minutes.

Cook Time: minutes

Ingredients:

- Lentils,rinsed
- Carrots,diced
- Celery,chopped
- Onion,diced
- Garlic,minced
- Vegetable broth
- Potatoes,cubed
- Butter or dairy-free spread.
- Plant-based milk, such as almond milk.

Instructions:

1. Preheat the oven to F (C).
2. In a large pot, sauté diced onion and minced garlic until fragrant.
3. Add diced carrots, chopped celery, rinsed lentils, and vegetable broth to the pot.

4. Simmer the lentil mixture until the vegetables are tender and the broth is absorbed.

5. Meanwhile, boil cubed potatoes until tender, then mash with butter, dairy-free spread, and plant-based milk.

6. Spread mashed potatoes over the lentil mixture in a baking dish.

7. Bake shepherd's pie in the oven for about minutes, or until the top turns golden brown.

8. Serve this vegetarian lentil shepherd's pie hot for a comforting and cancer-preventing dinner option!

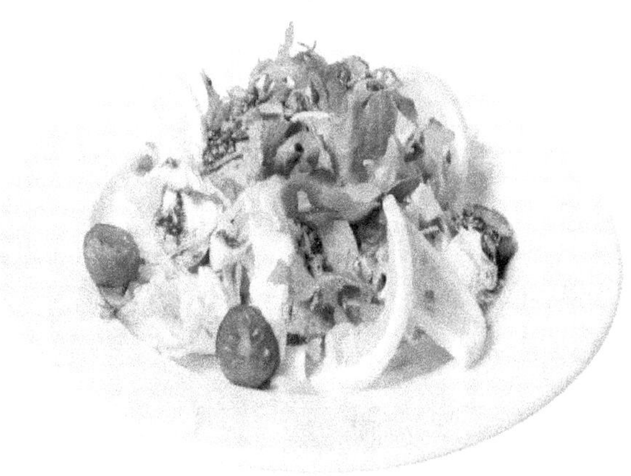

CHAPTER 6: SNACKS AND SIDES

Avocado and Chickpea Salad

This refreshing salad combines creamy avocado with protein-packed chickpeas, colorful veggies, and a zesty dressing for a nutritious and cancer-preventive snack or side dish.

Serving Size: 2

Prep Time: 10 minutes

Ingredients:

- Ripe avocado, diced
- Canned chickpeas, drained and rinsed
- Cherry tomatoes, halved
- Cucumber, diced
- Red onion, thinly sliced
- Fresh parsley, chopped
- Lemon juice, olive oil, salt, and pepper

Instructions:

1. In a large bowl, combine the diced avocado, chickpeas, cherry tomatoes, cucumber, red onion, and chopped parsley.
2. Drizzle with lemon juice and olive oil.
3. Season with salt and pepper to taste.
4. Toss gently to combine all ingredients.
5. Serve this avocado and chickpea salad chilled as a healthy and flavorful snack or side dish.

Roasted Beet Hummus

This vibrant hummus features roasted beets blended with chickpeas, garlic, and tahini for a colorful and cancer-preventive dip or spread.

 Serving Size: 6

Prep Time: 15 minutes

Cooking Time: 45 minutes

Ingredients:

- Beets, roasted and peeled

- Canned chickpeas,

- drained and rinsed

- Garlic cloves

- Tahini

- Lemon juice

- Cumin, salt, and pepper

Instructions:

1. Preheat the oven to 400°F (200°C).

2. Wrap beets in foil and roast until tender, about 45 minutes.

3. Peel the roasted beets and cut into chunks.

4. In a food processor, combine the roasted beets, chickpeas, garlic cloves, tahini, lemon juice, cumin, salt, and pepper.

5. Blend until smooth, adding water as needed for desired consistency.

6. Serve this roasted beet hummus with veggie sticks or whole grain crackers for a colorful and nutritious snack.

Quinoa and Black Bean Stuffed Bell Peppers

These colorful bell peppers are filled with protein-rich quinoa, black beans, corn, and spices for a satisfying and cancer-preventive snack or side dish.

Serving Size: 4

Prep Time: 20 minutes

Cooking Time: 30 minutes

Ingredients:

- Bell peppers (any color), halved and seeded
- Cooked quinoa
- Black beans, drained and rinsed
- Corn kernels (fresh or frozen)
- Salsa or diced tomatoes

- Mexican spices (cumin, chili powder)

Instructions:

1. Preheat the oven to 375°F (190°C).
2. In a bowl, mix together the cooked quinoa, black beans, corn kernels, salsa or diced tomatoes, and Mexican spices.
3. Stuff the halved bell peppers with the quinoa mixture.
4. Place the stuffed bell peppers in a baking dish and cover with foil.
5. Bake for about 25-30 minutes until the peppers are tender.
6. Serve these quinoa and black bean stuffed bell peppers as a wholesome snack or side dish.

Greek Yogurt Veggie Dip

This creamy dip features Greek yogurt blended with fresh herbs and veggies for a light and cancer-preventive option to pair with raw vegetables or whole grain crackers.

Serving Size: 4

Prep Time: 10 minutes

Ingredients:

- Greek yogurt
- Cucumber, grated and squeezed dry
- Dill or mint, chopped
- Lemon juice
- Garlic powder,
- salt, and pepper

Instructions:

1. In a bowl, mix together Greek yogurt, grated cucumber, chopped dill or mint, lemon juice, garlic powder, salt, and pepper.
2. Stir until well combined.
3. Chill the dip in the refrigerator for at least 30 minutes to allow flavors to meld.

4. Serve this Greek yogurt veggie dip with a platter of fresh vegetables for a light and refreshing snack or side dish.

Crispy Baked Kale Chips

These crunchy kale chips are seasoned with nutritional yeast and spices before being baked to perfection for a flavorful and cancer-preventive snack or side dish.

Serving Size: 2

Prep Time: 10 minutes

Cooking Time: 15 minutes

Ingredients:

- For Kale Chips
- Fresh kale leaves
- Olive oil
- Nutritional yeast
- Garlic powder
- Salt & pepper

Instructions:

1. Preheat oven to F (C).

2. Wash kale leaves & pat dry.

3. Tear kale leaves into bite-sized pieces & place in bowl.

4. Drizzle kale with olive oil & sprinkle with nutritional yeast,garlic powder,salt & pepper.

5. Toss kale until well coated.

6. Spread kale in single layer on baking sheet.

7. Bake kale chips in oven for about minutes or until crispy.

8. Serve these crispy baked kale chips hot as a nutritious & delicious snack or side dish!

Coconut Mango Chia Pudding

This tropical chia pudding features coconut milk,mango puree & chia seeds for creamy & cancer-preventive snack or dessert.

Serving Size: Makes about servings

Prep Time: minutes

Cooking Time: minutes

Ingredients:

- Coconut milk
- Mango,pureed
- Chia seeds
- Honey or maple syrup
- Vanilla extract

Instructions:

1. In bowl whisk together coconut milk,mango puree,chia seeds,honey or maple syrup & vanilla extract.
2. Cover bowl & refrigerate chia pudding for at least hours or overnight.
3. Stir pudding before serving & top with fresh mango slices & shredded coconut if desired.

4. Enjoy this coconut mango chia pudding as creamy & cancer-preventive snack or dessert!

Turmeric Roasted Cauliflower

This flavorful cauliflower is seasoned with turmeric,cumin & garlic before being roasted to crispy perfection for tasty & cancer-preventive snack or side dish.

Serving Size: Makes about servings
Prep Time: minutes
Cooking Time: minutes

Ingredients:
- Cauliflower florets
- Olive oil
- Turmeric
- Cumin
- Garlic powder
- Salt & pepper

Instructions:

1. Preheat oven to F (C).

2. In bowl toss cauliflower florets with olive oil,turmeric,cumin,garlic powder,salt & pepper until coated.

3. Spread cauliflower on baking sheet in single layer.

4. Roast cauliflower in oven for about minutes or until golden brown & crispy.

5. Serve this turmeric roasted cauliflower hot as flavorful & cancer-preventive snack or side dish!

Spinach and Feta Stuffed Mushrooms

These savory mushrooms are filled with spinach,feta cheese & herbs then baked to perfection for delicious & cancer-preventive snack or side dish.

Serving Size: Makes about servings

Prep Time: minutes

Cooking Time: minutes

Ingredients:

- Mushrooms,portobello or button
- Spinach,chopped
- Feta cheese
- Garlic,minced
- Fresh herbs (parsley,dill)
- Olive oil

Instructions:

1. Preheat oven to F (C).
2. Remove stems from mushrooms & place caps on baking sheet.
3. In skillet sauté chopped spinach,minced garlic,feta cheese,fresh herbs & olive oil until spinach is wilted.
4. Spoon spinach mixture into mushroom caps.
5. Bake stuffed mushrooms in oven for about minutes or until mushrooms are tender.

6. Serve these spinach & feta stuffed mushrooms hot as savory & cancer-preventive snack or side dish!

Baked Sweet Potato Fries

These crispy sweet potato fries are seasoned with paprika,cumin & garlic before being baked to perfection for tasty & cancer-preventive snack or side dish.

Serving Size: Makes about servings

Prep Time: minutes

Cooking Time: minutes

Ingredients:

- Sweet potatoes,julienned
- Olive oil
- Paprika
- Cumin
- Garlic powder
- Salt & pepper

Instructions:

1. Preheat oven to F (C).

2. In bowl toss julienned sweet potatoes with olive oil,paprika,cumin,garlic powder,salt & pepper until coated.

3. Spread sweet potatoes on baking sheet in single layer.

4. Bake sweet potato fries in oven for about minutes or until crispy.

5. Serve these baked sweet potato fries hot as flavorful & cancer-preventive snack or side dish!

Mediterranean Chickpea Salad

This vibrant salad features chickpeas,cucumbers,tomatoes,feta cheese & olives tossed in lemon-herb dressing for fresh & cancer-preventive snack or side dish.

Serving Size: Makes about servings

Prep Time: minutes

Cooking Time: minutes

Ingredients:

- Canned chickpeas,rinsed
- Cucumbers,diced
- Tomatoes,cherry or grape,halfed
- Feta cheese,cubed
- Kalamata olives,pitted
- Lemon juice
- Fresh herbs (parsley,dill)
- Olive oil
- Salt & pepper

Instructions:

1. In large bowl combine chickpeas,diced cucumbers,tomatoes,feta cheese,Kalamata olives,fresh herbs & lemon juice.
2. Drizzle salad with olive oil,salt & pepper then toss gently to combine all ingredients.

3. Chill salad in refrigerator for at least hour before serving.

4. Serve this Mediterranean chickpea salad cold as fresh & cancer-preventive snack or side dish!

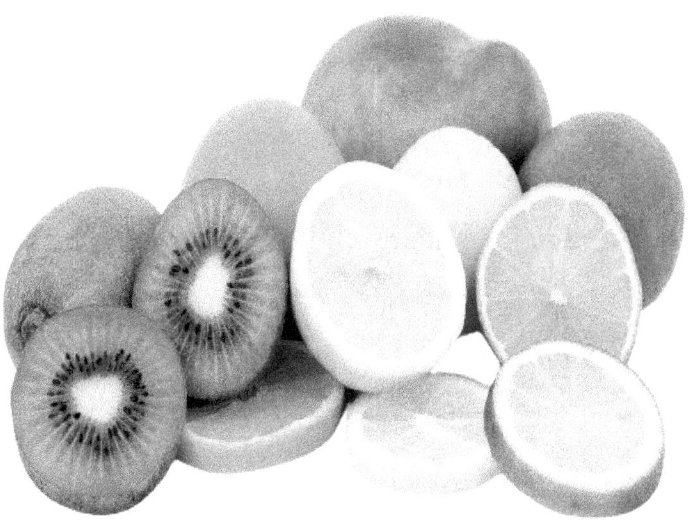

CHAPTER 7: DESSERTS AND TREATS

Berry Chia Seed Pudding

This antioxidant-rich chia seed pudding with mixed berries is a delicious and cancer-preventive dessert or snack.

Serving size: four.

Prep time: 10 minutes.

Cooking time: 4 hours (chill time)

Ingredients:

- Chia seeds.
- Almond Milk
- Mixed berries (strawberries, blueberries, raspberries) - Maple syrup or honey.
- Vanilla Extract

Instructions:

1. In a bowl, combine the chia seeds, almond milk, honey or maple syrup, and vanilla extract.
2. Stir in the mixed berries.
3. Cover and chill for at least 4 hours, or overnight.
4. Chill the berry chia seed pudding for a refreshing and cancer-preventive dessert.

Dark Chocolate Avocado Mousse

Combine ripe avocados with dark chocolate for a decadent and cancer-preventing treat.

Serving size: two.

Prep time: 15 minutes, cooking time: 0 minutes.

Ingredients:

- Ripe avocados.
- Dark chocolate chips.
- unsweetened cocoa powder.
- Honey, agave syrup

- Vanilla Extract

Instructions:

1. In a food processor, puree the avocados until smooth.
2. Melt the dark chocolate chips and mix with the avocado, cocoa powder, honey or agave syrup, and vanilla extract.
3. Blend until creamy and thoroughly combined.
4. Place the dark chocolate avocado mousse in the refrigerator for at least 30 minutes before serving.

Turmeric Golden Milk Popsicles

Infused with turmeric, ginger, and coconut milk, these frozen treats are both refreshing and cancer-preventive.

Serves 6 people - Takes 10 minutes to prepare.

Cooking Time: 4 hours (Freezing Time)

Ingredients:

- Coconut milk.

- Turmeric Powder

- Ginger Powder

- Cinnamon

- Honey or maple syrup.

Instructions:

1. In a bowl, combine the coconut milk, turmeric powder, ginger powder, cinnamon, and honey or maple syrup.

2. Pour the mixture into popsicle molds and insert the sticks.

3. Freeze for at least four hours, or until solid.

4. Enjoy these turmeric golden milk popsicles as a colorful and cancer-preventing dessert.

Matcha Green Tea Nice Cream

This dairy-free nice cream combines matcha green tea powder with frozen bananas to create a creamy and cancer-preventing dessert.

Serving size: two.

Prep time: 5 minutes, cooking time: 0 minutes.

Ingredients:

- Frozen bananas.
- Matcha Green Tea Powder
- Almond Milk
- Honey, agave syrup

Instructions:

1. In a blender, combine the frozen bananas, matcha green tea powder, almond milk, and honey/agave syrup.
2. Blend until smooth and creamy.

3. Serve the matcha green tea nice cream right away as a refreshing and cancer-preventive dessert.

Oatmeal Raisin Energy Bites

These no-bake energy bites contain oats, raisins, nuts, and seeds, making them a nutritious and cancer-preventing snack or dessert.

Serves 12 people - Takes 10 minutes to prepare - Cooks in 0 minutes

Ingredients:

- Rolled Oats
- Raisins
- almond butter and chia seeds.
- Honey or maple syrup.

Instructions:

1. In a bowl, combine the rolled oats, raisins, almond butter, chia seeds, and honey or maple syrup.

2. Form the mixture into bite-size balls.

3. Place the oatmeal raisin energy bites in the refrigerator for at least 30 minutes before serving.

Coconut Almond Bliss Balls

This sweet and cancer-preventive treat combines coconut, almonds, dates, and cacao.

Serves 10 people - Takes 15 minutes to prepare.

Cooking time: 0 minutes.

Ingredients:

- Shredded coconut.
- almonds, dates,
- cacao powder,
- vanilla extract,

instructions:

1. In a food processor, combine shredded coconut, almonds, dates, cacao powder, and vanilla extract until the mixture holds together.

2. Form the mixture into small balls.

3. Refrigerate the coconut almond bliss balls for a quick and delicious cancer-prevention snack or dessert.

Pumpkin Spice Chia Pudding

This festive chia pudding is flavored with pumpkin puree and warm spices such as cinnamon and nutmeg for a comforting and cancer-preventive dessert or snack.

Service Size: Makes about servings

Preparation Time: minutes.

Cooking Time: hours (Chilling Time)

Ingredients:

- Chia seeds

- Almond milk

- Pumpkin puree

- Maple syrup

- Cinnamon

- Nutmeg

Instructions:

1. In a bowl, combine the chia seeds, almond milk, pumpkin puree, maple syrup, cinnamon, and nutmeg.

2. Cover the bowl and refrigerate the chia pudding for at least an hour or overnight.

3. Before serving, stir the pudding and top with more cinnamon, if desired.

4. Enjoy this pumpkin spice chia pudding as a comforting, cancer-preventing dessert or snack!

Blueberry Yogurt Parfait

This colorful parfait combines Greek yogurt, fresh blueberries, honey, and granola for a light, cancer-preventing dessert or snack.

Service Size: Makes about servings.
Preparation Time: minutes.
Cook Time: minutes

Ingredients:

- Greek yogurt.
- Blueberries
- Honey
- Granola

Instructions:

1. In a glass, layer Greek yogurt, fresh blueberries, honey, and granola.

2. Repeat layers until the glass is full, ending with granola on top.

3. Serve this blueberry yogurt parfait cold for a light and cancer-preventing dessert or snack!

Cinnamon Apple Crisp

This warm apple crisp, spiced with cinnamon and topped with oat crumble, is a comforting and cancer-preventing dessert.

Service Size: Makes about servings.

Preparation Time: minutes.

Cook Time: minutes

Ingredients:

- Apples,sliced
- Cinnamon
- Oats
- Flour
- Butter

- Honey

Instructions:

1. Preheat the oven to F (C).

2. Toss sliced apples with cinnamon in a bowl until evenly coated, then transfer to a baking dish.

3. In a separate bowl, combine oats, flour, butter, and honey until crumbly; then sprinkle over apples.

4. Bake apple crisp in the oven for about minutes, or until the topping is golden brown and the apples are soft.

5. Serve this cinnamon apple crisp warm for a comforting and cancer-preventing dessert!

Coconut Mango Sorbet

This tropical sorbet combines ripe mangoes and coconut milk for a creamy, cancer-preventing frozen treat.

Service Size: Makes about servings.

Preparation Time: minutes.

Cook Time: minutes

Ingredients:

- Mangoes,pureed
- Coconut Milk
- Honey, maple syrup
- Lime Juice
- Shredded coconut (optional)

Instructions:

1. In a blender, combine mango puree, coconut milk, honey or maple syrup, and lime juice. Blend until smooth.

2. Pour the mango mixture into a shallow dish and freeze for hours, or until set.

3. Allow the sorbet to soften at room temperature for a few minutes before scooping it into bowls.

4. Top with shredded coconut if desired, and enjoy this creamy, cancer-preventing frozen treat!

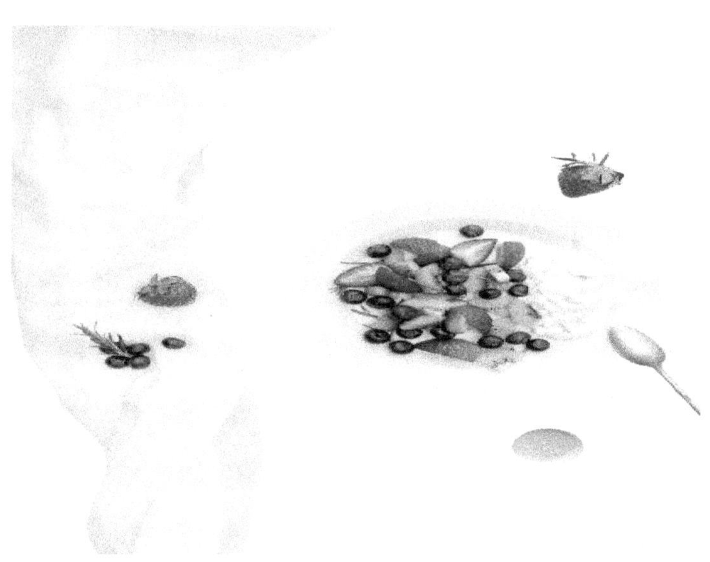

CHAPTER8 : BONUS 7-DAY MEAL PLANNING

In today's world, where health and wellness are top priorities, taking a mindful approach to meal planning can be an effective tool for promoting overall well-being. One important aspect of this is to incorporate cancer prevention recipes into our daily diets. We can prevent cancer by focusing on nutrient-rich foods and ingredients known for their cancer-fighting properties. In this comprehensive guide, we'll look at a 7-day meal plan full of delicious and nutritious recipes to help you prioritize your health and well-being.

Day 1: Begin your week with a vibrant Berry Blast Smoothie Bowl. This antioxidant-rich bowl includes berries, spinach, and chia seeds, making it a tasty and nutritious way to start the day.

Day 2: Turmeric Roasted Vegetables are a colorful and flavorful dish full of anti-inflammatory benefits. Roast a variety of vegetables with turmeric for a tasty and nutritious meal.

Day 3: Lentil and Vegetable Soup is a hearty and comforting meal full of plant-based protein and fiber. This nutrient-dense soup is ideal for nourishing the body and promoting overall health.

Day 4: For dinner, try grilled salmon with lemon dill sauce. Salmon is high in omega-3 fatty acids, which have been associated with a lower risk of cancer. Serve it with roasted asparagus for a light and flavorful meal.

Day 5: For a plant-based dinner, try Chickpea and Spinach Curry. This fragrant and flavorful dish contains cancer-fighting spices such as turmeric, cumin, and coriander.

Day 6 - Quinoa Stuffed Bell peppers are a colorful and nutritionally dense meal option. Fill bell peppers with quinoa, black beans, and corn for a hearty and nutritious dinner.

Day 7: Finish the week on a sweet note with Mixed Berry Chia Seed Pudding. Chia seeds contain omega-3 fatty acids and fiber, making this dessert both tasty and nutritious.

Following this 7-day meal plan, which includes cancer prevention recipes, allows you to nourish your body with wholesome ingredients while also taking proactive steps to reduce your cancer risk. Accept the power of food to promote health and well-being, one delicious meal at a time. Begin planning your week with these engaging and nutritious recipes, and embark on a journey to a healthier, more vibrant you.

CONCLUSION

Additional Resources

addition to the previously mentioned 7-day meal plan, there are numerous resources that provide a wealth of recipes and information on cancer prevention through nutrition. Here are some other resources where you can find delicious and nutritious recipes to help you achieve your health goals:

1. Cookbooks: There are several cookbooks that focus on cancer prevention and support through healthy eating. Look for titles like Rebecca Katz's "The Cancer-Fighting Kitchen," Ann Ogden Gaffney's "Cook for Your Life," and Dr. David Servan-Schreiber's "Anti-Cancer Cookbook." These books include a variety of recipes for nourishing and supporting your body during and after cancer treatment.

2. Websites and Blogs: Many websites and blogs focus on providing recipes and resources for cancer prevention through nutrition. Websites such as the American Institute for Cancer Research (AICR), Cancer Council Australia, and the World Cancer Research Fund provide a variety of healthy recipes, meal plans, and nutritional information focused on cancer prevention.

3. Nutrition Apps: There are several nutrition apps available to help you track your food intake, plan meals, and discover new cancer-prevention recipes. Apps like MyFitnessPal, Lose It!, and Fooducate provide recipe suggestions, meal planning tools, and nutritional advice to help you make informed dietary decisions.

4. Social Media: Instagram, Pinterest, and Facebook all have accounts and pages dedicated to sharing healthy cancer prevention recipes. Follow influencers, nutritionists, and oncology nutrition organizations to get new ideas and inspiration for incorporating nutrient-dense foods into your daily diet.

5. Community Resources: Local community centers, cancer support groups, and hospitals frequently offer cooking classes, workshops, and events centered on cancer prevention nutrition. These resources can help you gain hands-on experience, expert advice, and a supportive environment for learning how to prepare healthy meals that promote overall wellness.

6. Nutrition Workshops and Seminars: Keep an eye out for upcoming workshops, seminars, and webinars hosted by registered dietitians, nutritionists, and healthcare professionals who specialize in oncology nutrition. These events provide useful information, practical tips, and evidence-based recommendations for including cancer-fighting foods in your diet.

By exploring these additional resources and seeking expert advice, you can broaden your understanding of nutrition for cancer prevention and discover a variety of recipes and meal ideas to help you on your health journey. Remember that even minor changes to your diet can have a significant impact on your overall well-being, so continue to prioritize your health and seek out resources that will help you make informed decisions for a healthier lifestyle.